A Universal Food Diary

A 12-Week Diet Journal and Food Tracker for Almost Any Diet

Practical Journals and Diaries

FTL Publications
Minnetonka, Minnesota

FTL Publications
P O Box 1363
Minnetonka, MN 55345-0363
www.ftlpublications.com
mail@ftlpublications.com

Cover photo © natuska106 - Fotolia.com

Printed in the United States of America

ISBN 978-1-936881-42-0

How to Use this Food Diary

This food diary is adaptable to almost any kind of diet. Whether you're counting calories, fat, fiber, carbs, sodium, etc, there are spaces for them. You only need use the spaces you're tracking.

Food	Amount	Calories	Fat	Fiber	Carbs	Sodium	
nonfat milk	*1 cup*	*86*					

The last column is blank so that you can fill in any other value you're keeping track of.

For example:

Food	Amount	Calories	Fat	Fiber	Carbs	Sodium	*Protein*
nonfat milk	*1 cup*	*86*					*8.35 g*

There are also checkoff spaces for dairy servings, water, and fruits/vegetables. If you find there are items that you want to check off and there isn't a specific space for them, just use the last few lines of the page.

For example:

Grains	X	X					
Healthy oils	X	X	X				

At the beginning of each week, there is a page to record measurements, goals for the week, and what you're going to do for fun. (Yes, have some fun! Unless you do something you enjoy every day, your weight loss efforts will get boring and tedious.)

There's a wealth of information plus nutritional guidelines at ChooseMyPlate.gov, which has lots of useful resources no matter what diet plan you follow...all free! (See summary next page.)

Consult a medical professional before starting any weight loss plan.

EAT THE MYPLATE WAY

Enjoy your food but eat less.

Avoid oversized portions.

Make half your plate fruits and vegetables.

Make at least half your grains whole.

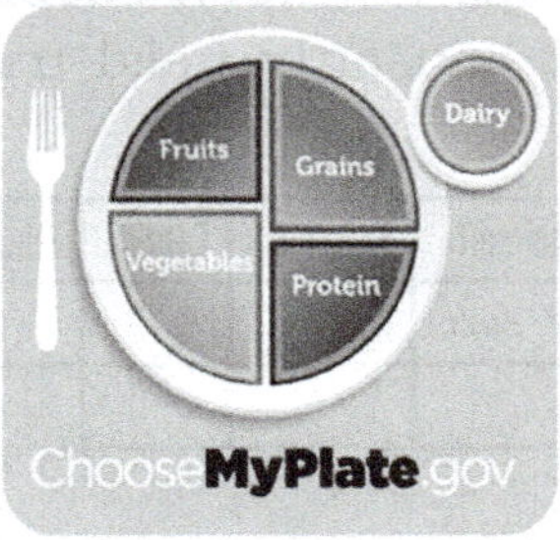

Compare sodium in foods like soup, bread, and frozen meals and choose foods with lower numbers.

Drink water instead of sugary drinks.

Switch to fat-free or low-fat (1%) milk.

Be active your way.

HOW TO FILL MY PLATE

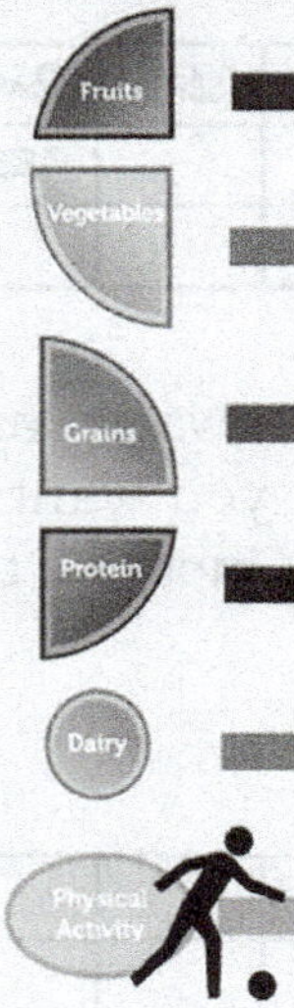

- **Fruits:** Apples, Bananas, Grapefruit, Lemons, Oranges, Strawberries, Cantaloupe, 100% Apple Juice, 100% Grape Juice
- **Vegetables:** Dark Green Leafy Lettuce, Broccoli, Potatoes, Corn, Butternut Squash, Red Pepper, Garbanzo Beans, Zucchini
- **Grains:** Brown Rice, Rolled Oats, Popcorn, Whole-Wheat Flour, Whole-Wheat Spaghetti, Bulgur, Whole Rye, Quinoa
- **Protein:** Lean Cuts of Beef, Pork, Chcken, Eggs, Black Beans, Lentils, Soy Beans, Almonds, Walnuts, Haddock, Salmon, Shrimp, Tuna
- **Dairy:** Fat-Free or Low-Fat (1%) Milk, Yogurt, and Cheese, Calcium-Fortified Soy Milk
- **Physical Activity:** Walking, Jogging, Biking, Hiking, Tennis, Basketball, Soccer, Swimming

GET STARTED!

1

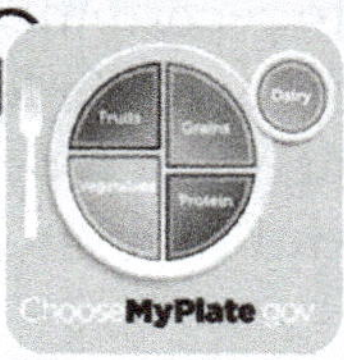

Use ChooseMyPlate.gov for health tips and resources.

2

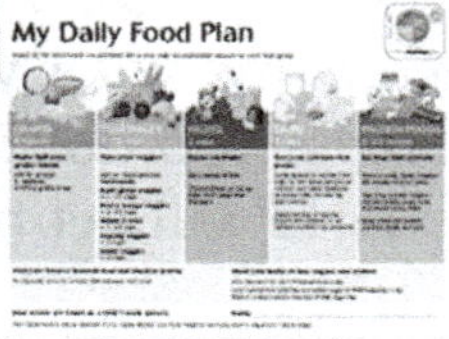

Select your daily food plan on ChooseMyPlate.gov. Use it as a guide to building a healthy plate.

3

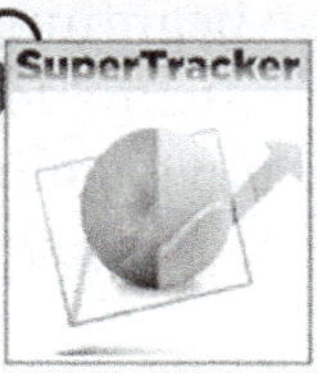

Determine how many calories you should consume per day using SuperTracker.usda.gov

USDA United States Department of Agriculture

Center for Nutrition Policy and Promotion
USDA is an equal opportunity provider and employer.

Beginning of the Week Statistics

(Track any or all of the items below)

Measurements	Today	Last Week	Difference
Weight			
Bust/Chest			
Waist			
Hips			
Arms			
Legs			

Goals for this week:

What I'm doing for fun this week:

Notes:

Date:

Food	Amount	Calories	Fat	Fiber	Carbs	Sodium	

Dairy ☐ ☐ ☐ Three 8 oz. glasses of milk, or servings of cheese, yogurt, etc.

Water ☐ ☐ ☐ ☐ ☐ ☐ ☐ ☐ Up to eight 8 oz. servings

Fruits/Vegetables ☐ ☐ ☐ ☐ ☐ ☐ ☐ ☐ ☐ Up to 9 half-cup servings

Activity		**Mood**	

Date:

Food	Amount	Calories	Fat	Fiber	Carbs	Sodium	

Dairy ☐☐☐ Three 8 oz. glasses of milk, or servings of cheese, yogurt, etc.

Water ☐☐☐☐☐☐☐☐ Up to eight 8 oz. servings

Fruits/Vegetables ☐☐☐☐☐☐☐☐☐ Up to 9 half-cup servings

Activity ______ **Mood** ______

Date:

Food	Amount	Calories	Fat	Fiber	Carbs	Sodium	

Dairy ☐☐☐ Three 8 oz. glasses of milk, or servings of cheese, yogurt, etc.

Water ☐☐☐☐☐☐☐☐ Up to eight 8 oz. servings

Fruits/Vegetables ☐☐☐☐☐☐☐☐☐ Up to 9 half-cup servings

Activity ____________ **Mood** ____________

Date:

Food	Amount	Calories	Fat	Fiber	Carbs	Sodium	

Dairy ☐☐☐ Three 8 oz. glasses of milk, or servings of cheese, yogurt, etc.

Water ☐☐☐☐☐☐☐☐ Up to eight 8 oz. servings

Fruits/Vegetables ☐☐☐☐☐☐☐☐☐ Up to 9 half-cup servings

Activity ____________ **Mood** ____________

Date:

Food	Amount	Calories	Fat	Fiber	Carbs	Sodium	

Dairy ☐ ☐ ☐ Three 8 oz. glasses of milk, or servings of cheese, yogurt, etc.

Water ☐ ☐ ☐ ☐ ☐ ☐ ☐ ☐ Up to eight 8 oz. servings

Fruits/Vegetables ☐ ☐ ☐ ☐ ☐ ☐ ☐ ☐ ☐ Up to 9 half-cup servings

Activity ______ **Mood** ______

Date:

Food	Amount	Calories	Fat	Fiber	Carbs	Sodium	

Dairy ☐☐☐ Three 8 oz. glasses of milk, or servings of cheese, yogurt, etc.

Water ☐☐☐☐☐☐☐☐ Up to eight 8 oz. servings

Fruits/Vegetables ☐☐☐☐☐☐☐☐☐ Up to 9 half-cup servings

Activity		**Mood**	

Date:

Food	Amount	Calories	Fat	Fiber	Carbs	Sodium	

Dairy Three 8 oz. glasses of milk, or servings of cheese, yogurt, etc.

Water Up to eight 8 oz. servings

Fruits/Vegetables Up to 9 half-cup servings

Activity **Mood**

Beginning of the Week Statistics

Measurements	Today	Last Week	Difference
Weight			
Bust/Chest			
Waist			
Hips			
Arms			
Legs			

Goals for this week:

What I'm doing for fun this week:

Notes:

Date:

Food	Amount	Calories	Fat	Fiber	Carbs	Sodium	

Dairy ☐☐☐ Three 8 oz. glasses of milk, or servings of cheese, yogurt, etc.

Water ☐☐☐☐☐☐☐☐ Up to eight 8 oz. servings

Fruits/Vegetables ☐☐☐☐☐☐☐☐☐ Up to 9 half-cup servings

Activity | **Mood**

Date:

Food	Amount	Calories	Fat	Fiber	Carbs	Sodium	

Dairy	☐ ☐ ☐	Three 8 oz. glasses of milk, or servings of cheese, yogurt, etc.
Water	☐ ☐ ☐ ☐ ☐ ☐ ☐ ☐	Up to eight 8 oz. servings
Fruits/Vegetables	☐ ☐ ☐ ☐ ☐ ☐ ☐ ☐ ☐	Up to 9 half-cup servings
Activity		**Mood**

Date:

Food	Amount	Calories	Fat	Fiber	Carbs	Sodium	

Dairy ☐☐☐ Three 8 oz. glasses of milk, or servings of cheese, yogurt, etc.

Water ☐☐☐☐☐☐☐☐ Up to eight 8 oz. servings

Fruits/Vegetables ☐☐☐☐☐☐☐☐☐ Up to 9 half-cup servings

Activity ______ **Mood** ______

Date:

Food	Amount	Calories	Fat	Fiber	Carbs	Sodium	

Dairy				Three 8 oz. glasses of milk, or servings of cheese, yogurt, etc.					
Water									Up to eight 8 oz. servings
Fruits/Vegetables										Up to 9 half-cup servings

Activity		**Mood**	

Date:

Food	Amount	Calories	Fat	Fiber	Carbs	Sodium	

Dairy ☐☐☐ Three 8 oz. glasses of milk, or servings of cheese, yogurt, etc.

Water ☐☐☐☐☐☐☐☐ Up to eight 8 oz. servings

Fruits/Vegetables ☐☐☐☐☐☐☐☐☐ Up to 9 half-cup servings

Activity | **Mood**

Date:

Food	Amount	Calories	Fat	Fiber	Carbs	Sodium	

Dairy ☐☐☐ Three 8 oz. glasses of milk, or servings of cheese, yogurt, etc.

Water ☐☐☐☐☐☐☐☐ Up to eight 8 oz. servings

Fruits/Vegetables ☐☐☐☐☐☐☐☐☐ Up to 9 half-cup servings

Activity   **Mood**

Date:

Food	Amount	Calories	Fat	Fiber	Carbs	Sodium	

Dairy				Three 8 oz. glasses of milk, or servings of cheese, yogurt, etc.						
Water									Up to eight 8 oz. servings	
Fruits/Vegetables										Up to 9 half-cup servings
Activity		**Mood**								

Beginning of the Week Statistics

Measurements	Today	Last Week	Difference
Weight			
Bust/Chest			
Waist			
Hips			
Arms			
Legs			

Goals for this week:

What I'm doing for fun this week:

Notes:

Date:

Food	Amount	Calories	Fat	Fiber	Carbs	Sodium	

Dairy ☐ ☐ ☐ Three 8 oz. glasses of milk, or servings of cheese, yogurt, etc.

Water ☐ ☐ ☐ ☐ ☐ ☐ ☐ ☐ Up to eight 8 oz. servings

Fruits/Vegetables ☐ ☐ ☐ ☐ ☐ ☐ ☐ ☐ ☐ Up to 9 half-cup servings

Activity | **Mood**

Date:

Food	Amount	Calories	Fat	Fiber	Carbs	Sodium	

Dairy ☐☐☐ Three 8 oz. glasses of milk, or servings of cheese, yogurt, etc.

Water ☐☐☐☐☐☐☐☐ Up to eight 8 oz. servings

Fruits/Vegetables ☐☐☐☐☐☐☐☐☐ Up to 9 half-cup servings

Activity | **Mood**

Date:

Food	Amount	Calories	Fat	Fiber	Carbs	Sodium	

Dairy ☐☐☐ Three 8 oz. glasses of milk, or servings of cheese, yogurt, etc.

Water ☐☐☐☐☐☐☐☐ Up to eight 8 oz. servings

Fruits/Vegetables ☐☐☐☐☐☐☐☐☐ Up to 9 half-cup servings

Activity ____________ **Mood** ____________

Date:

Food	Amount	Calories	Fat	Fiber	Carbs	Sodium	

Dairy				Three 8 oz. glasses of milk, or servings of cheese, yogurt, etc.					
Water									Up to eight 8 oz. servings
Fruits/Vegetables										Up to 9 half-cup servings

Activity		**Mood**	

Date:

Food	Amount	Calories	Fat	Fiber	Carbs	Sodium	

Dairy ☐☐☐ Three 8 oz. glasses of milk, or servings of cheese, yogurt, etc.

Water ☐☐☐☐☐☐☐☐ Up to eight 8 oz. servings

Fruits/Vegetables ☐☐☐☐☐☐☐☐☐ Up to 9 half-cup servings

Activity ________ **Mood** ________

Date:

Food	Amount	Calories	Fat	Fiber	Carbs	Sodium	

Dairy ☐ ☐ ☐ Three 8 oz. glasses of milk, or servings of cheese, yogurt, etc.

Water ☐ ☐ ☐ ☐ ☐ ☐ ☐ ☐ Up to eight 8 oz. servings

Fruits/Vegetables ☐ ☐ ☐ ☐ ☐ ☐ ☐ ☐ ☐ Up to 9 half-cup servings

Activity   **Mood**

Date:

Food	Amount	Calories	Fat	Fiber	Carbs	Sodium	

Dairy ☐☐☐ Three 8 oz. glasses of milk, or servings of cheese, yogurt, etc.

Water ☐☐☐☐☐☐☐☐ Up to eight 8 oz. servings

Fruits/Vegetables ☐☐☐☐☐☐☐☐☐ Up to 9 half-cup servings

Activity | **Mood**

Beginning of the Week Statistics

Measurements	Today	Last Week	Difference
Weight			
Bust/Chest			
Waist			
Hips			
Arms			
Legs			

Goals for this week:

What I'm doing for fun this week:

Notes:

Date:

Food	Amount	Calories	Fat	Fiber	Carbs	Sodium	

Dairy ☐ ☐ ☐ Three 8 oz. glasses of milk, or servings of cheese, yogurt, etc.

Water ☐ ☐ ☐ ☐ ☐ ☐ ☐ ☐ Up to eight 8 oz. servings

Fruits/Vegetables ☐ ☐ ☐ ☐ ☐ ☐ ☐ ☐ ☐ Up to 9 half-cup servings

Activity | **Mood**

Date:

Food	Amount	Calories	Fat	Fiber	Carbs	Sodium	

Dairy ☐☐☐ Three 8 oz. glasses of milk, or servings of cheese, yogurt, etc.

Water ☐☐☐☐☐☐☐☐ Up to eight 8 oz. servings

Fruits/Vegetables ☐☐☐☐☐☐☐☐☐ Up to 9 half-cup servings

Activity | **Mood**

Date:

Food	Amount	Calories	Fat	Fiber	Carbs	Sodium	

Dairy				Three 8 oz. glasses of milk, or servings of cheese, yogurt, etc.						
Water									Up to eight 8 oz. servings	
Fruits/Vegetables										Up to 9 half-cup servings

Activity ____ **Mood** ____

Date:

Food	Amount	Calories	Fat	Fiber	Carbs	Sodium	

Dairy ☐ ☐ ☐ Three 8 oz. glasses of milk, or servings of cheese, yogurt, etc.

Water ☐ ☐ ☐ ☐ ☐ ☐ ☐ ☐ Up to eight 8 oz. servings

Fruits/Vegetables ☐ ☐ ☐ ☐ ☐ ☐ ☐ ☐ ☐ Up to 9 half-cup servings

Activity ______ **Mood** ______

Date:

Food	Amount	Calories	Fat	Fiber	Carbs	Sodium	

Dairy ☐☐☐ Three 8 oz. glasses of milk, or servings of cheese, yogurt, etc.

Water ☐☐☐☐☐☐☐☐ Up to eight 8 oz. servings

Fruits/Vegetables ☐☐☐☐☐☐☐☐☐ Up to 9 half-cup servings

Activity   **Mood**

Date:

Food	Amount	Calories	Fat	Fiber	Carbs	Sodium	

Dairy ☐ ☐ ☐ Three 8 oz. glasses of milk, or servings of cheese, yogurt, etc.

Water ☐ ☐ ☐ ☐ ☐ ☐ ☐ ☐ Up to eight 8 oz. servings

Fruits/Vegetables ☐ ☐ ☐ ☐ ☐ ☐ ☐ ☐ ☐ Up to 9 half-cup servings

Activity ____________ **Mood** ____________

Date:

Food	Amount	Calories	Fat	Fiber	Carbs	Sodium	

Dairy ☐☐☐ Three 8 oz. glasses of milk, or servings of cheese, yogurt, etc.

Water ☐☐☐☐☐☐☐☐ Up to eight 8 oz. servings

Fruits/Vegetables ☐☐☐☐☐☐☐☐☐ Up to 9 half-cup servings

Activity ______ **Mood** ______

Beginning of the Week Statistics

Measurements	Today	Last Week	Difference
Weight			
Bust/Chest			
Waist			
Hips			
Arms			
Legs			

Goals for this week:

What I'm doing for fun this week:

Notes:

Date:

Food	Amount	Calories	Fat	Fiber	Carbs	Sodium	

Dairy ☐☐☐ Three 8 oz. glasses of milk, or servings of cheese, yogurt, etc.

Water ☐☐☐☐☐☐☐☐ Up to eight 8 oz. servings

Fruits/Vegetables ☐☐☐☐☐☐☐☐☐ Up to 9 half-cup servings

Activity | **Mood**

Date:

Food	Amount	Calories	Fat	Fiber	Carbs	Sodium	

Dairy ☐☐☐ Three 8 oz. glasses of milk, or servings of cheese, yogurt, etc.

Water ☐☐☐☐☐☐☐☐ Up to eight 8 oz. servings

Fruits/Vegetables ☐☐☐☐☐☐☐☐☐ Up to 9 half-cup servings

Activity | **Mood**

Date:

Food	Amount	Calories	Fat	Fiber	Carbs	Sodium	

Dairy ☐☐☐ Three 8 oz. glasses of milk, or servings of cheese, yogurt, etc.

Water ☐☐☐☐☐☐☐☐ Up to eight 8 oz. servings

Fruits/Vegetables ☐☐☐☐☐☐☐☐☐ Up to 9 half-cup servings

Activity ____ **Mood** ____

Date:

Food	Amount	Calories	Fat	Fiber	Carbs	Sodium	

Dairy ☐☐☐ Three 8 oz. glasses of milk, or servings of cheese, yogurt, etc.

Water ☐☐☐☐☐☐☐☐ Up to eight 8 oz. servings

Fruits/Vegetables ☐☐☐☐☐☐☐☐☐ Up to 9 half-cup servings

Activity ____________ **Mood** ____________

Date:

Food	Amount	Calories	Fat	Fiber	Carbs	Sodium	

Dairy				Three 8 oz. glasses of milk, or servings of cheese, yogurt, etc.						
Water									Up to eight 8 oz. servings	
Fruits/Vegetables										Up to 9 half-cup servings
Activity		**Mood**								

Date:

Food	Amount	Calories	Fat	Fiber	Carbs	Sodium	

Dairy				Three 8 oz. glasses of milk, or servings of cheese, yogurt, etc.					
Water									Up to eight 8 oz. servings
Fruits/Vegetables										Up to 9 half-cup servings

Activity		**Mood**	

Date:

Food	Amount	Calories	Fat	Fiber	Carbs	Sodium	

Dairy				Three 8 oz. glasses of milk, or servings of cheese, yogurt, etc.						
Water									Up to eight 8 oz. servings	
Fruits/Vegetables										Up to 9 half-cup servings
Activity					**Mood**					

Beginning of the Week Statistics

Measurements	Today	Last Week	Difference
Weight			
Bust/Chest			
Waist			
Hips			
Arms			
Legs			

Goals for this week:

What I'm doing for fun this week:

Notes:

Date:

Food	Amount	Calories	Fat	Fiber	Carbs	Sodium	

Dairy ☐ ☐ ☐ Three 8 oz. glasses of milk, or servings of cheese, yogurt, etc.

Water ☐ ☐ ☐ ☐ ☐ ☐ ☐ ☐ Up to eight 8 oz. servings

Fruits/Vegetables ☐ ☐ ☐ ☐ ☐ ☐ ☐ ☐ ☐ Up to 9 half-cup servings

Activity | **Mood**

Date:

Food	Amount	Calories	Fat	Fiber	Carbs	Sodium	

Dairy					Three 8 oz. glasses of milk, or servings of cheese, yogurt, etc.

Water									Up to eight 8 oz. servings

Fruits/Vegetables										Up to 9 half-cup servings

Activity		Mood	

Date:

Food	Amount	Calories	Fat	Fiber	Carbs	Sodium	

Dairy ☐ ☐ ☐ Three 8 oz. glasses of milk, or servings of cheese, yogurt, etc.

Water ☐ ☐ ☐ ☐ ☐ ☐ ☐ ☐ Up to eight 8 oz. servings

Fruits/Vegetables ☐ ☐ ☐ ☐ ☐ ☐ ☐ ☐ ☐ Up to 9 half-cup servings

Activity ______ **Mood** ______

Date:

Food	Amount	Calories	Fat	Fiber	Carbs	Sodium	

Dairy				Three 8 oz. glasses of milk, or servings of cheese, yogurt, etc.						
Water									Up to eight 8 oz. servings	
Fruits/Vegetables										Up to 9 half-cup servings

Activity		**Mood**	

Date:

Food	Amount	Calories	Fat	Fiber	Carbs	Sodium	

Dairy				Three 8 oz. glasses of milk, or servings of cheese, yogurt, etc.

Water									Up to eight 8 oz. servings

Fruits/Vegetables										Up to 9 half-cup servings

Activity		**Mood**	

Date:

Food	Amount	Calories	Fat	Fiber	Carbs	Sodium	

Dairy ☐☐☐ Three 8 oz. glasses of milk, or servings of cheese, yogurt, etc.

Water ☐☐☐☐☐☐☐☐ Up to eight 8 oz. servings

Fruits/Vegetables ☐☐☐☐☐☐☐☐☐ Up to 9 half-cup servings

Activity _______________ **Mood** _______________

Date:

Food	Amount	Calories	Fat	Fiber	Carbs	Sodium	

Dairy ☐☐☐ Three 8 oz. glasses of milk, or servings of cheese, yogurt, etc.

Water ☐☐☐☐☐☐☐☐ Up to eight 8 oz. servings

Fruits/Vegetables ☐☐☐☐☐☐☐☐☐ Up to 9 half-cup servings

Activity | **Mood**

Beginning of the Week Statistics

Measurements	Today	Last Week	Difference
Weight			
Bust/Chest			
Waist			
Hips			
Arms			
Legs			

Goals for this week:

What I'm doing for fun this week:

Notes:

Date:

Food	Amount	Calories	Fat	Fiber	Carbs	Sodium	

Dairy ☐☐☐ Three 8 oz. glasses of milk, or servings of cheese, yogurt, etc.

Water ☐☐☐☐☐☐☐☐ Up to eight 8 oz. servings

Fruits/Vegetables ☐☐☐☐☐☐☐☐☐ Up to 9 half-cup servings

Activity ____________ **Mood** ____________

Date:

Food	Amount	Calories	Fat	Fiber	Carbs	Sodium	

Dairy Three 8 oz. glasses of milk, or servings of cheese, yogurt, etc.

Water Up to eight 8 oz. servings

Fruits/Vegetables Up to 9 half-cup servings

Activity **Mood**

Date:

Food	Amount	Calories	Fat	Fiber	Carbs	Sodium	

Dairy ☐☐☐ Three 8 oz. glasses of milk, or servings of cheese, yogurt, etc.

Water ☐☐☐☐☐☐☐☐ Up to eight 8 oz. servings

Fruits/Vegetables ☐☐☐☐☐☐☐☐☐ Up to 9 half-cup servings

Activity | **Mood**

Date:

Food	Amount	Calories	Fat	Fiber	Carbs	Sodium	

Dairy ☐☐☐ Three 8 oz. glasses of milk, or servings of cheese, yogurt, etc.

Water ☐☐☐☐☐☐☐☐ Up to eight 8 oz. servings

Fruits/Vegetables ☐☐☐☐☐☐☐☐☐ Up to 9 half-cup servings

Activity   **Mood**

Date:

Food	Amount	Calories	Fat	Fiber	Carbs	Sodium	

Dairy ☐☐☐ Three 8 oz. glasses of milk, or servings of cheese, yogurt, etc.

Water ☐☐☐☐☐☐☐☐ Up to eight 8 oz. servings

Fruits/Vegetables ☐☐☐☐☐☐☐☐☐ Up to 9 half-cup servings

Activity ____________ **Mood** ____________

Date:

Food	Amount	Calories	Fat	Fiber	Carbs	Sodium	

Dairy				Three 8 oz. glasses of milk, or servings of cheese, yogurt, etc.						
Water									Up to eight 8 oz. servings	
Fruits/Vegetables										Up to 9 half-cup servings

Activity		**Mood**	

Date:

Food	Amount	Calories	Fat	Fiber	Carbs	Sodium	

Dairy				Three 8 oz. glasses of milk, or servings of cheese, yogurt, etc.						
Water									Up to eight 8 oz. servings	
Fruits/Vegetables										Up to 9 half-cup servings

Activity		**Mood**	

Beginning of the Week Statistics

Measurements	Today	Last Week	Difference
Weight			
Bust/Chest			
Waist			
Hips			
Arms			
Legs			

Goals for this week:

What I'm doing for fun this week:

Notes:

Date:

Food	Amount	Calories	Fat	Fiber	Carbs	Sodium	

Dairy ☐ ☐ ☐ Three 8 oz. glasses of milk, or servings of cheese, yogurt, etc.

Water ☐ ☐ ☐ ☐ ☐ ☐ ☐ ☐ Up to eight 8 oz. servings

Fruits/Vegetables ☐ ☐ ☐ ☐ ☐ ☐ ☐ ☐ ☐ Up to 9 half-cup servings

Activity | **Mood**

Date:

Food	Amount	Calories	Fat	Fiber	Carbs	Sodium	

Dairy ☐☐☐ Three 8 oz. glasses of milk, or servings of cheese, yogurt, etc.

Water ☐☐☐☐☐☐☐☐ Up to eight 8 oz. servings

Fruits/Vegetables ☐☐☐☐☐☐☐☐☐ Up to 9 half-cup servings

Activity | **Mood**

Date:

Food	Amount	Calories	Fat	Fiber	Carbs	Sodium	

Dairy ☐☐☐ Three 8 oz. glasses of milk, or servings of cheese, yogurt, etc.

Water ☐☐☐☐☐☐☐☐ Up to eight 8 oz. servings

Fruits/Vegetables ☐☐☐☐☐☐☐☐☐ Up to 9 half-cup servings

Activity **Mood**

Date:

Food	Amount	Calories	Fat	Fiber	Carbs	Sodium	

Dairy ☐☐☐ Three 8 oz. glasses of milk, or servings of cheese, yogurt, etc.

Water ☐☐☐☐☐☐☐☐ Up to eight 8 oz. servings

Fruits/Vegetables ☐☐☐☐☐☐☐☐☐ Up to 9 half-cup servings

Activity | **Mood**

Date:

Food	Amount	Calories	Fat	Fiber	Carbs	Sodium	

Dairy ☐☐☐ Three 8 oz. glasses of milk, or servings of cheese, yogurt, etc.

Water ☐☐☐☐☐☐☐☐ Up to eight 8 oz. servings

Fruits/Vegetables ☐☐☐☐☐☐☐☐☐ Up to 9 half-cup servings

Activity		**Mood**	

Date:

Food	Amount	Calories	Fat	Fiber	Carbs	Sodium	

Dairy				Three 8 oz. glasses of milk, or servings of cheese, yogurt, etc.						
Water									Up to eight 8 oz. servings	
Fruits/Vegetables										Up to 9 half-cup servings

Activity		**Mood**	

Date:

Food	Amount	Calories	Fat	Fiber	Carbs	Sodium	

Dairy ☐☐☐ Three 8 oz. glasses of milk, or servings of cheese, yogurt, etc.

Water ☐☐☐☐☐☐☐☐ Up to eight 8 oz. servings

Fruits/Vegetables ☐☐☐☐☐☐☐☐☐ Up to 9 half-cup servings

Activity | **Mood**

Beginning of the Week Statistics

Measurements	Today	Last Week	Difference
Weight			
Bust/Chest			
Waist			
Hips			
Arms			
Legs			

Goals for this week:

What I'm doing for fun this week:

Notes:

Date:

Food	Amount	Calories	Fat	Fiber	Carbs	Sodium	

Dairy				Three 8 oz. glasses of milk, or servings of cheese, yogurt, etc.						
Water									Up to eight 8 oz. servings	
Fruits/Vegetables										Up to 9 half-cup servings

Activity		**Mood**	

Date:

Food	Amount	Calories	Fat	Fiber	Carbs	Sodium	

Dairy ☐☐☐ Three 8 oz. glasses of milk, or servings of cheese, yogurt, etc.

Water ☐☐☐☐☐☐☐☐ Up to eight 8 oz. servings

Fruits/Vegetables ☐☐☐☐☐☐☐☐☐ Up to 9 half-cup servings

Activity		**Mood**	

Date:

Food	Amount	Calories	Fat	Fiber	Carbs	Sodium	

Dairy ☐ ☐ ☐ Three 8 oz. glasses of milk, or servings of cheese, yogurt, etc.

Water ☐ ☐ ☐ ☐ ☐ ☐ ☐ ☐ Up to eight 8 oz. servings

Fruits/Vegetables ☐ ☐ ☐ ☐ ☐ ☐ ☐ ☐ ☐ Up to 9 half-cup servings

Activity		**Mood**	

Date:

Food	Amount	Calories	Fat	Fiber	Carbs	Sodium	

Dairy ☐☐☐ Three 8 oz. glasses of milk, or servings of cheese, yogurt, etc.

Water ☐☐☐☐☐☐☐☐ Up to eight 8 oz. servings

Fruits/Vegetables ☐☐☐☐☐☐☐☐☐ Up to 9 half-cup servings

Activity | **Mood**

Date:

Food	Amount	Calories	Fat	Fiber	Carbs	Sodium	

Dairy ☐☐☐ Three 8 oz. glasses of milk, or servings of cheese, yogurt, etc.

Water ☐☐☐☐☐☐☐☐ Up to eight 8 oz. servings

Fruits/Vegetables ☐☐☐☐☐☐☐☐☐ Up to 9 half-cup servings

Activity		**Mood**	

Date:

Food	Amount	Calories	Fat	Fiber	Carbs	Sodium	

Dairy				Three 8 oz. glasses of milk, or servings of cheese, yogurt, etc.

Water									Up to eight 8 oz. servings

Fruits/Vegetables										Up to 9 half-cup servings

Activity		**Mood**	

Date:

Food	Amount	Calories	Fat	Fiber	Carbs	Sodium	

Dairy				Three 8 oz. glasses of milk, or servings of cheese, yogurt, etc.					
Water									Up to eight 8 oz. servings
Fruits/Vegetables										Up to 9 half-cup servings

Activity		**Mood**	

Beginning of the Week Statistics

Measurements	Today	Last Week	Difference
Weight			
Bust/Chest			
Waist			
Hips			
Arms			
Legs			

Goals for this week:

What I'm doing for fun this week:

Notes:

Date:

Food	Amount	Calories	Fat	Fiber	Carbs	Sodium	

Dairy ☐☐☐ Three 8 oz. glasses of milk, or servings of cheese, yogurt, etc.

Water ☐☐☐☐☐☐☐☐ Up to eight 8 oz. servings

Fruits/Vegetables ☐☐☐☐☐☐☐☐☐ Up to 9 half-cup servings

Activity		**Mood**	

Date:

Food	Amount	Calories	Fat	Fiber	Carbs	Sodium	

Dairy ☐☐☐ Three 8 oz. glasses of milk, or servings of cheese, yogurt, etc.

Water ☐☐☐☐☐☐☐☐ Up to eight 8 oz. servings

Fruits/Vegetables ☐☐☐☐☐☐☐☐☐ Up to 9 half-cup servings

Activity   **Mood**

Date:

Food	Amount	Calories	Fat	Fiber	Carbs	Sodium	

Dairy ☐ ☐ ☐ Three 8 oz. glasses of milk, or servings of cheese, yogurt, etc.

Water ☐ ☐ ☐ ☐ ☐ ☐ ☐ ☐ Up to eight 8 oz. servings

Fruits/Vegetables ☐ ☐ ☐ ☐ ☐ ☐ ☐ ☐ ☐ Up to 9 half-cup servings

Activity | **Mood**

Date:

Food	Amount	Calories	Fat	Fiber	Carbs	Sodium	

Dairy ☐☐☐ Three 8 oz. glasses of milk, or servings of cheese, yogurt, etc.

Water ☐☐☐☐☐☐☐☐ Up to eight 8 oz. servings

Fruits/Vegetables ☐☐☐☐☐☐☐☐☐ Up to 9 half-cup servings

Activity | **Mood**

Date:

Food	Amount	Calories	Fat	Fiber	Carbs	Sodium	

Dairy ☐ ☐ ☐ Three 8 oz. glasses of milk, or servings of cheese, yogurt, etc.

Water ☐ ☐ ☐ ☐ ☐ ☐ ☐ ☐ Up to eight 8 oz. servings

Fruits/Vegetables ☐ ☐ ☐ ☐ ☐ ☐ ☐ ☐ ☐ Up to 9 half-cup servings

Activity   **Mood**

Date:

Food	Amount	Calories	Fat	Fiber	Carbs	Sodium	

Dairy ☐☐☐ Three 8 oz. glasses of milk, or servings of cheese, yogurt, etc.

Water ☐☐☐☐☐☐☐☐ Up to eight 8 oz. servings

Fruits/Vegetables ☐☐☐☐☐☐☐☐☐ Up to 9 half-cup servings

Activity ______ **Mood** ______

Date:

Food	Amount	Calories	Fat	Fiber	Carbs	Sodium	

Dairy ☐ ☐ ☐ Three 8 oz. glasses of milk, or servings of cheese, yogurt, etc.

Water ☐ ☐ ☐ ☐ ☐ ☐ ☐ ☐ Up to eight 8 oz. servings

Fruits/Vegetables ☐ ☐ ☐ ☐ ☐ ☐ ☐ ☐ ☐ Up to 9 half-cup servings

Activity   **Mood**

Beginning of the Week Statistics

Measurements	Today	Last Week	Difference
Weight			
Bust/Chest			
Waist			
Hips			
Arms			
Legs			

Goals for this week:

What I'm doing for fun this week:

Notes:

Date:

Food	Amount	Calories	Fat	Fiber	Carbs	Sodium	

Dairy ☐☐☐ Three 8 oz. glasses of milk, or servings of cheese, yogurt, etc.

Water ☐☐☐☐☐☐☐☐ Up to eight 8 oz. servings

Fruits/Vegetables ☐☐☐☐☐☐☐☐☐ Up to 9 half-cup servings

Activity | **Mood**

Date:

Food	Amount	Calories	Fat	Fiber	Carbs	Sodium	

Dairy				Three 8 oz. glasses of milk, or servings of cheese, yogurt, etc.

Water									Up to eight 8 oz. servings

Fruits/Vegetables										Up to 9 half-cup servings

Activity		**Mood**	

Date:

Food	Amount	Calories	Fat	Fiber	Carbs	Sodium	

Dairy ☐ ☐ ☐ Three 8 oz. glasses of milk, or servings of cheese, yogurt, etc.

Water ☐ ☐ ☐ ☐ ☐ ☐ ☐ ☐ Up to eight 8 oz. servings

Fruits/Vegetables ☐ ☐ ☐ ☐ ☐ ☐ ☐ ☐ ☐ Up to 9 half-cup servings

Activity		**Mood**	

Date:

Food	Amount	Calories	Fat	Fiber	Carbs	Sodium	

Dairy ☐ ☐ ☐ Three 8 oz. glasses of milk, or servings of cheese, yogurt, etc.

Water ☐ ☐ ☐ ☐ ☐ ☐ ☐ ☐ Up to eight 8 oz. servings

Fruits/Vegetables ☐ ☐ ☐ ☐ ☐ ☐ ☐ ☐ ☐ Up to 9 half-cup servings

Activity ______ **Mood** ______

Date:

Food	Amount	Calories	Fat	Fiber	Carbs	Sodium	

Dairy ☐☐☐ Three 8 oz. glasses of milk, or servings of cheese, yogurt, etc.

Water ☐☐☐☐☐☐☐☐ Up to eight 8 oz. servings

Fruits/Vegetables ☐☐☐☐☐☐☐☐☐ Up to 9 half-cup servings

Activity		**Mood**	

Date:

Food	Amount	Calories	Fat	Fiber	Carbs	Sodium	

Dairy ☐ ☐ ☐ Three 8 oz. glasses of milk, or servings of cheese, yogurt, etc.

Water ☐ ☐ ☐ ☐ ☐ ☐ ☐ ☐ Up to eight 8 oz. servings

Fruits/Vegetables ☐ ☐ ☐ ☐ ☐ ☐ ☐ ☐ ☐ Up to 9 half-cup servings

Activity		**Mood**	

Date:

Food	Amount	Calories	Fat	Fiber	Carbs	Sodium	

Dairy ☐☐☐ Three 8 oz. glasses of milk, or servings of cheese, yogurt, etc.

Water ☐☐☐☐☐☐☐☐ Up to eight 8 oz. servings

Fruits/Vegetables ☐☐☐☐☐☐☐☐☐ Up to 9 half-cup servings

Activity | **Mood**

Beginning of the Week Statistics

Measurements	Today	Last Week	Difference
Weight			
Bust/Chest			
Waist			
Hips			
Arms			
Legs			

Goals for this week:

What I'm doing for fun this week:

Notes:

Date:

Food	Amount	Calories	Fat	Fiber	Carbs	Sodium	

Dairy ☐☐☐ Three 8 oz. glasses of milk, or servings of cheese, yogurt, etc.

Water ☐☐☐☐☐☐☐☐ Up to eight 8 oz. servings

Fruits/Vegetables ☐☐☐☐☐☐☐☐☐ Up to 9 half-cup servings

Activity ______ **Mood** ______

Date:

Food	Amount	Calories	Fat	Fiber	Carbs	Sodium	

Dairy ☐ ☐ ☐ Three 8 oz. glasses of milk, or servings of cheese, yogurt, etc.

Water ☐ ☐ ☐ ☐ ☐ ☐ ☐ ☐ Up to eight 8 oz. servings

Fruits/Vegetables ☐ ☐ ☐ ☐ ☐ ☐ ☐ ☐ ☐ Up to 9 half-cup servings

Activity ______ **Mood** ______

Date:

Food	Amount	Calories	Fat	Fiber	Carbs	Sodium	

Dairy ☐☐☐ Three 8 oz. glasses of milk, or servings of cheese, yogurt, etc.

Water ☐☐☐☐☐☐☐☐ Up to eight 8 oz. servings

Fruits/Vegetables ☐☐☐☐☐☐☐☐☐ Up to 9 half-cup servings

Activity		**Mood**	

Date:

Food	Amount	Calories	Fat	Fiber	Carbs	Sodium	

Dairy				Three 8 oz. glasses of milk, or servings of cheese, yogurt, etc.						
Water									Up to eight 8 oz. servings	
Fruits/Vegetables										Up to 9 half-cup servings

Activity		**Mood**	

Date:

Food	Amount	Calories	Fat	Fiber	Carbs	Sodium	

Dairy				Three 8 oz. glasses of milk, or servings of cheese, yogurt, etc.

Water									Up to eight 8 oz. servings

Fruits/Vegetables										Up to 9 half-cup servings

Activity		**Mood**	

Date:

Food	Amount	Calories	Fat	Fiber	Carbs	Sodium	

Dairy ☐ ☐ ☐ Three 8 oz. glasses of milk, or servings of cheese, yogurt, etc.

Water ☐ ☐ ☐ ☐ ☐ ☐ ☐ ☐ Up to eight 8 oz. servings

Fruits/Vegetables ☐ ☐ ☐ ☐ ☐ ☐ ☐ ☐ ☐ Up to 9 half-cup servings

Activity		Mood	

Date:

Food	Amount	Calories	Fat	Fiber	Carbs	Sodium	

Dairy				Three 8 oz. glasses of milk, or servings of cheese, yogurt, etc.

Water									Up to eight 8 oz. servings

Fruits/Vegetables										Up to 9 half-cup servings

Activity		**Mood**	

Made in the USA
Monee, IL
04 November 2026

67377448R00056